Jack's Diabetes

by
William G. Bentrim
Illustrated by
AcesGraphics

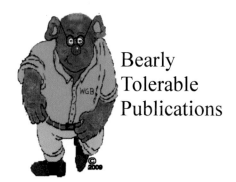

Bearly
Tolerable
Publications

Author's Note

Children have many mysteries that they courageously face on a daily basis. One of my goals in writing is to demystify or explain to children the basis for some of the confusing situations in their lives.

This book's goal is to help children realize that although the onset of diabetes can be frightening it does not mean the cessation of normal life. I have used the insulin pump as an example of how insulin can be delivered to treat diabetes. The pump is only one method that can be used to treat diabetes. Online reports indicate that many pump users feel that the pump provides them with a better quality of life than alternative therapies. I am not recommending the insulin pump nor am I a doctor. My goal is to provide a story that helps both the youthful diabetic and their peers to understand the impact of diabetes and one method of therapy. It is not a recommendation for that therapy and all medical decisions should be discussed with your physician.

—-Bill

ISBN-13: 978-1475268331
ISBN-10: 1475268335

Cover art and illustrations by AcesGraphics

Kudos to my wife for her patience and perseverance and to Barbara Smith my editor and also to J. the young man who was kind enough to share his thoughts on his diabetes. I would also like to thank Patricia A. Trymbiski, DNP, CDE, BC-ADM, of the Doylestown Hospital Diabetes Center for her technical expertise in helping me to hopefully avoid a faux pax in my diabetes description.

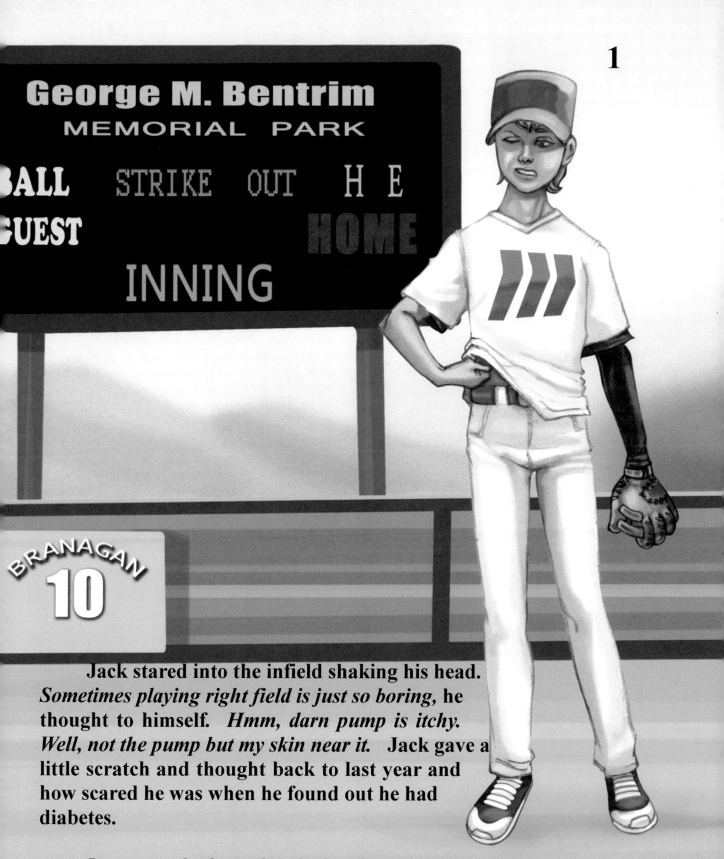

Jack stared into the infield shaking his head. *Sometimes playing right field is just so boring,* he thought to himself. *Hmm, darn pump is itchy. Well, not the pump but my skin near it.* Jack gave a little scratch and thought back to last year and how scared he was when he found out he had diabetes.

I sure am lucky to be playing baseball, he thought.

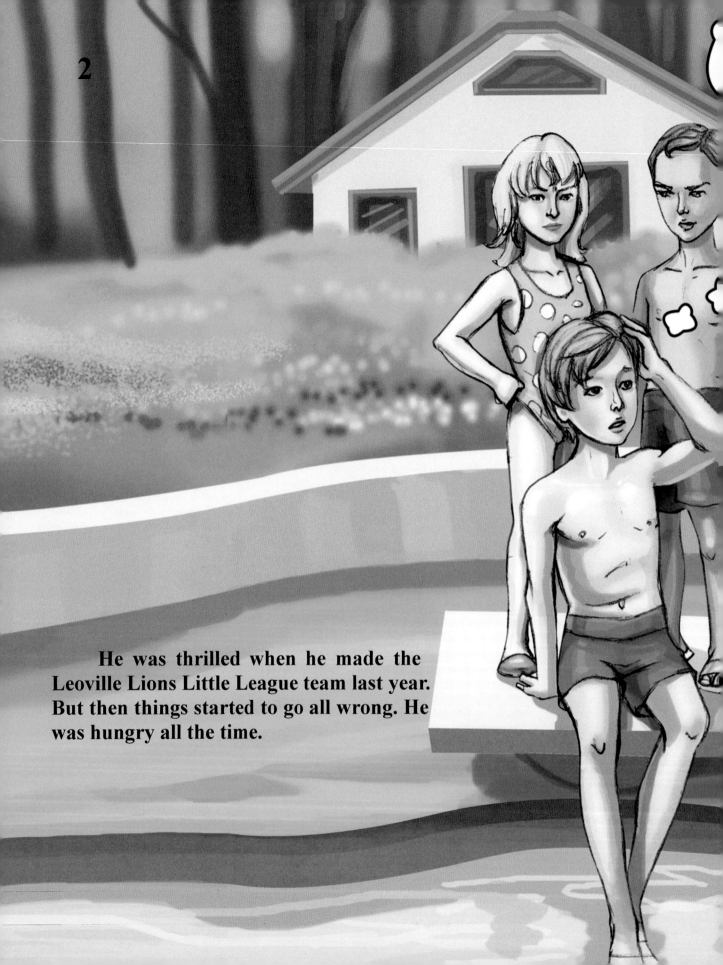

He was thrilled when he made the Leoville Lions Little League team last year. But then things started to go all wrong. He was hungry all the time.

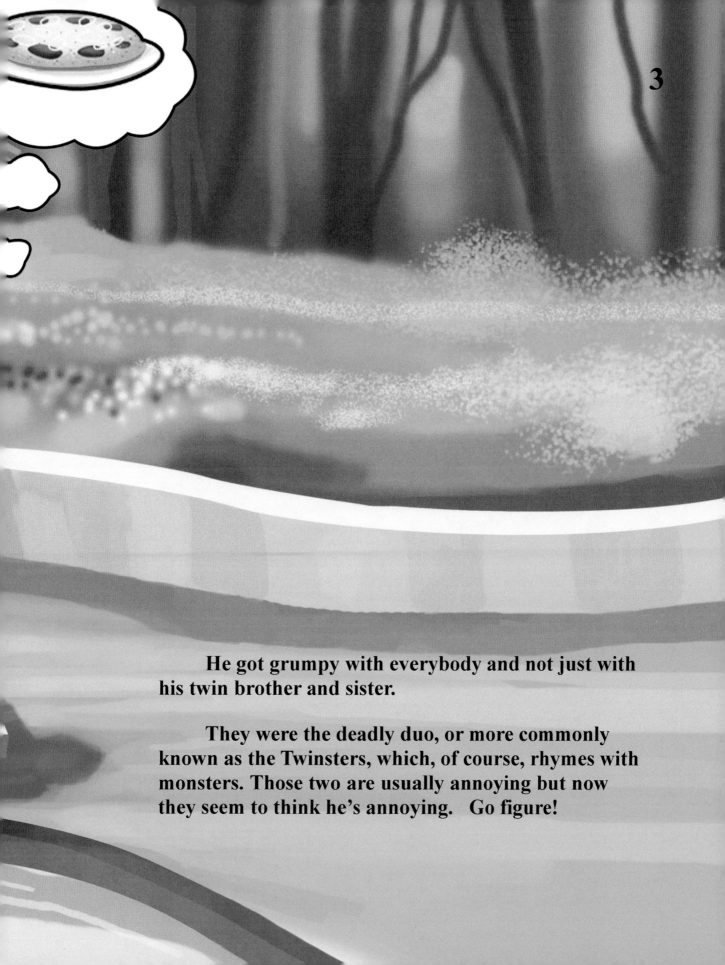

He got grumpy with everybody and not just with his twin brother and sister.

They were the deadly duo, or more commonly known as the Twinsters, which, of course, rhymes with monsters. Those two are usually annoying but now they seem to think he's annoying.   Go figure!

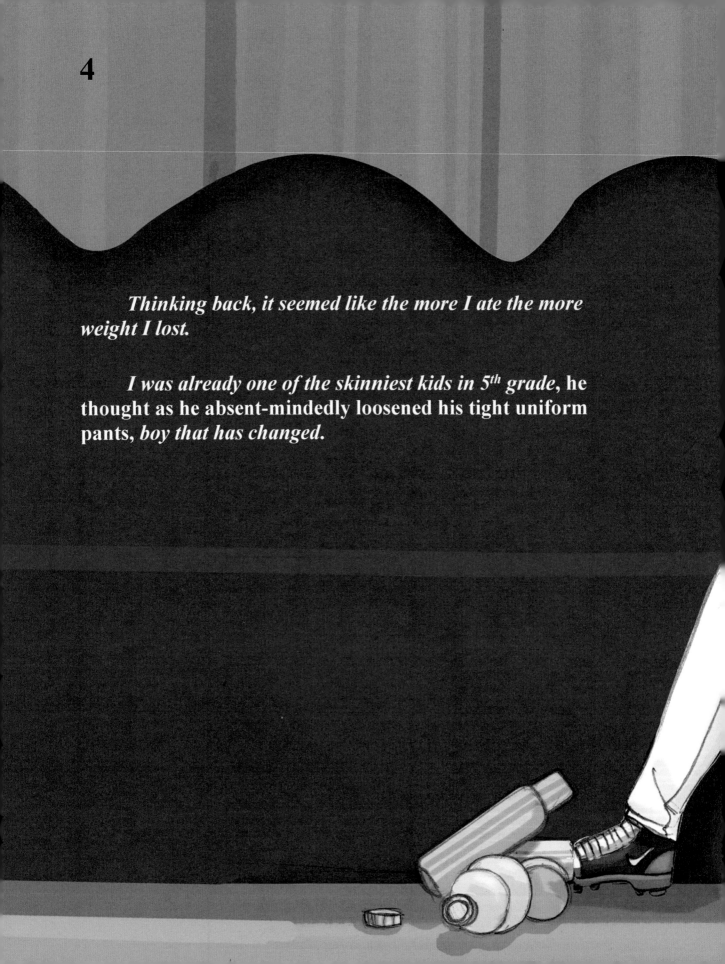

Thinking back, it seemed like the more I ate the more weight I lost.

I was already one of the skinniest kids in 5th grade, he thought as he absent-mindedly loosened his tight uniform pants, *boy that has changed.*

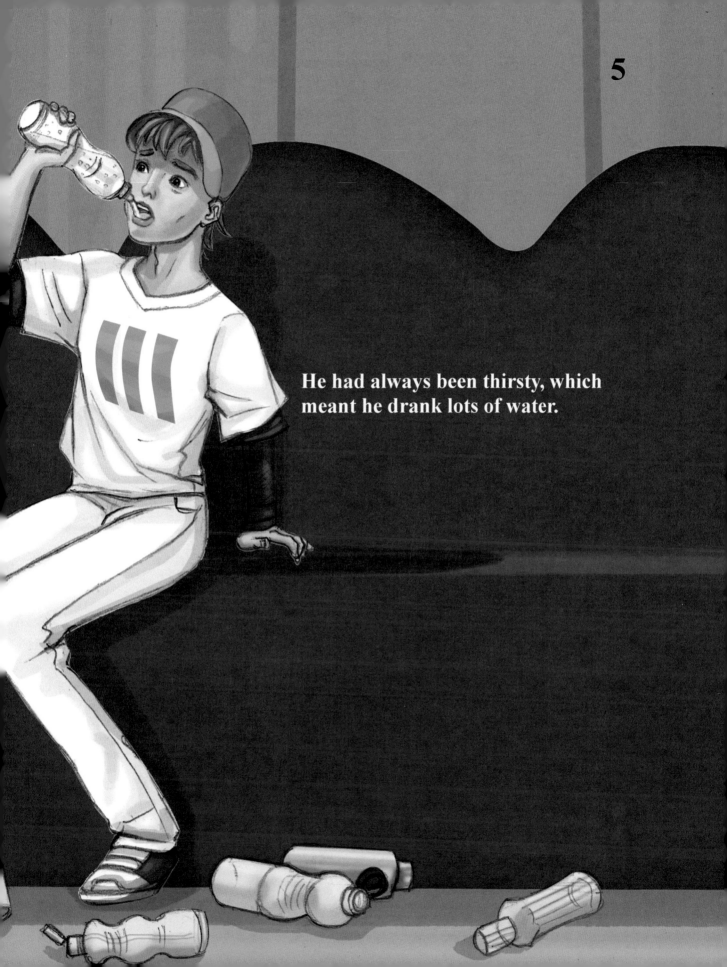

He had always been thirsty, which meant he drank lots of water.

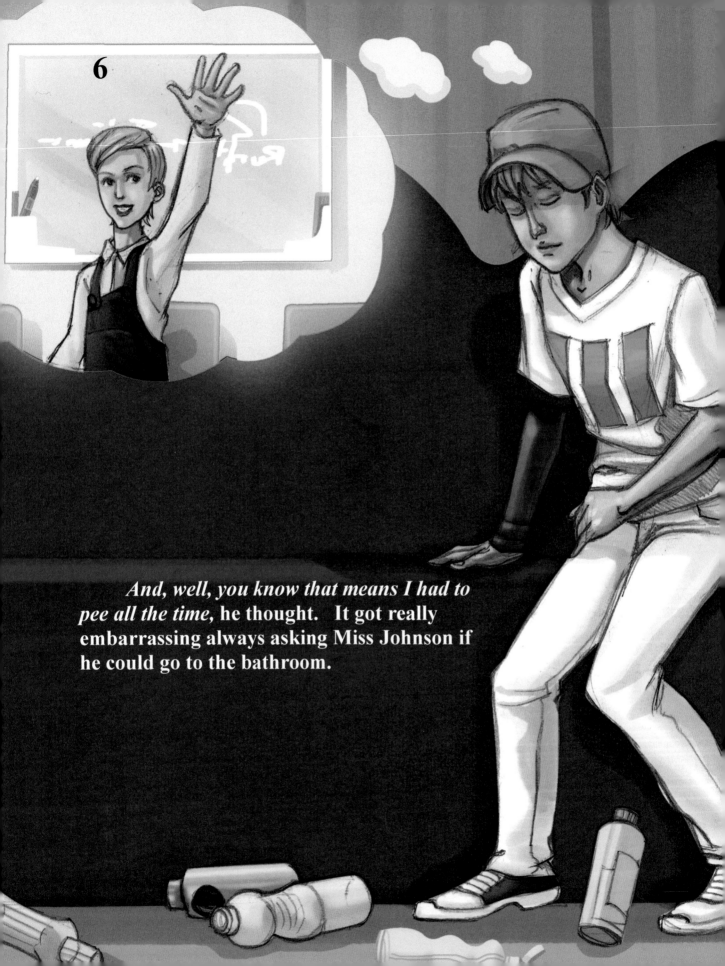

6

And, well, you know that means I had to pee all the time, he thought. It got really embarrassing always asking Miss Johnson if he could go to the bathroom.

Then baseball started to slip, he thought. *I was just too darn tired most of the time.*

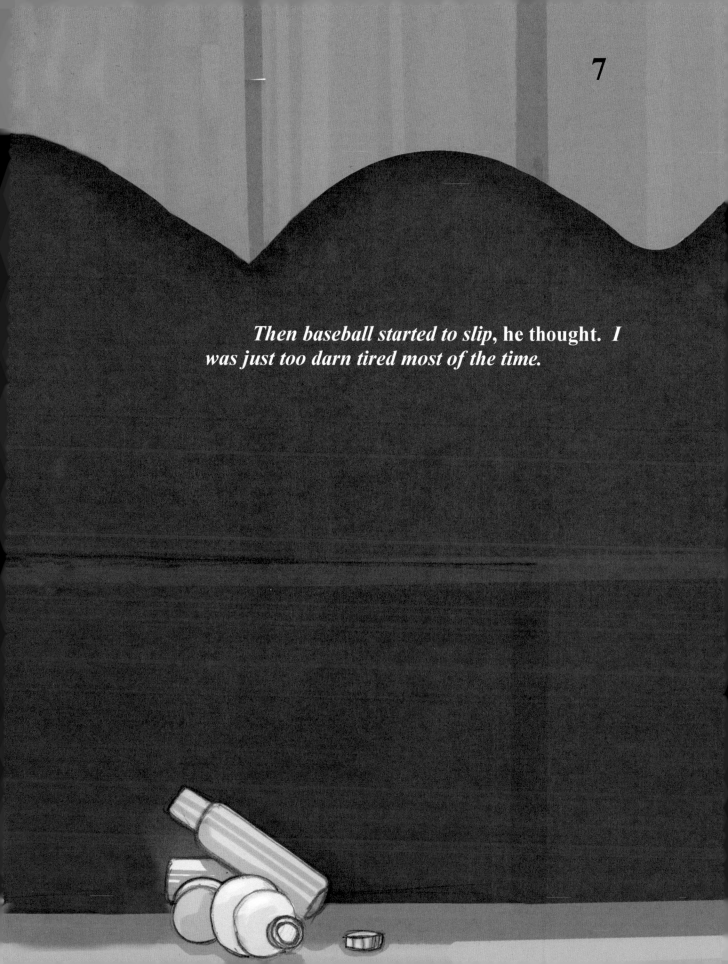

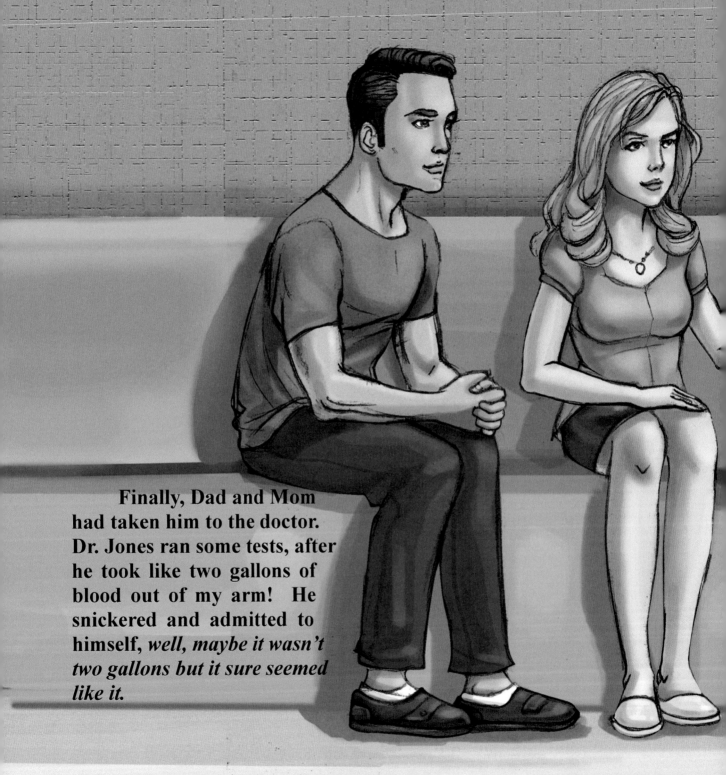

Finally, Dad and Mom had taken him to the doctor. Dr. Jones ran some tests, after he took like two gallons of blood out of my arm! He snickered and admitted to himself, *well, maybe it wasn't two gallons but it sure seemed like it.*

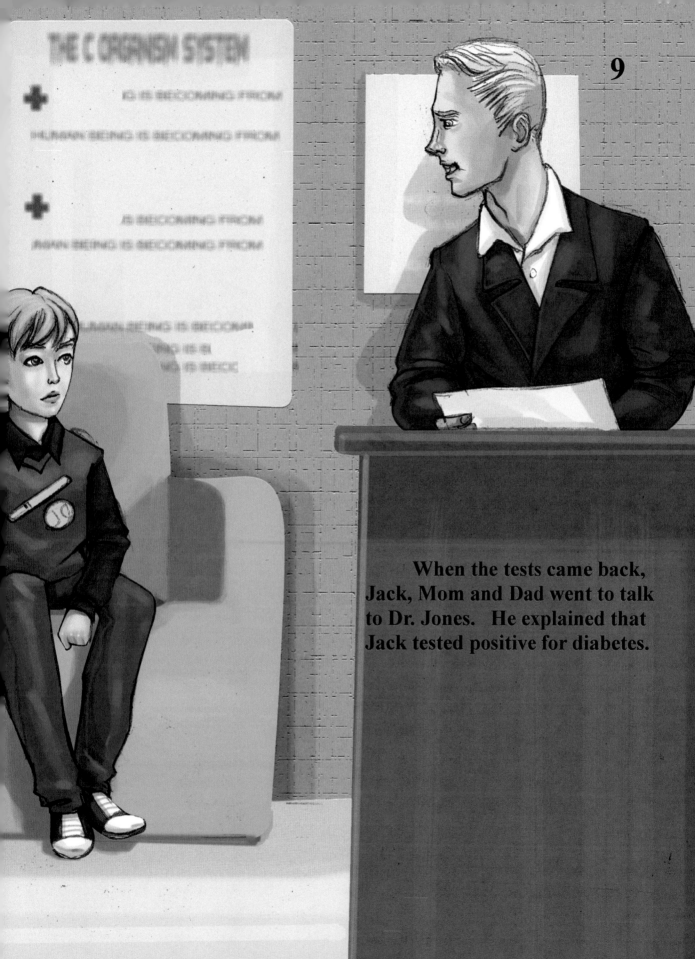

When the tests came back, Jack, Mom and Dad went to talk to Dr. Jones. He explained that Jack tested positive for diabetes.

10

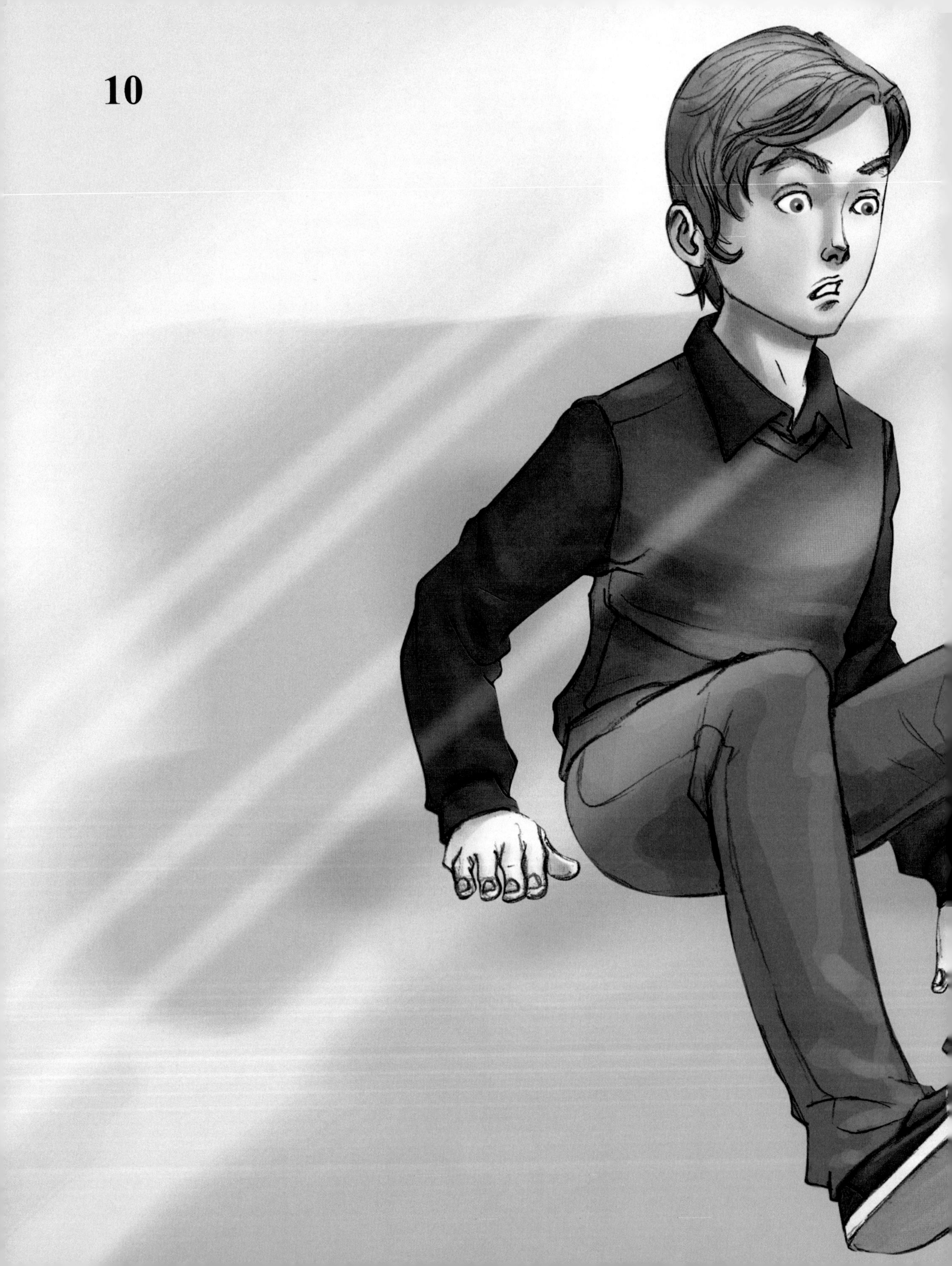

Jack had thought that couldn't be right! Grandpa had diabetes and it has something to do with sugar. Besides Grandpa was old!

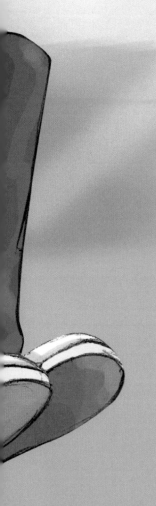

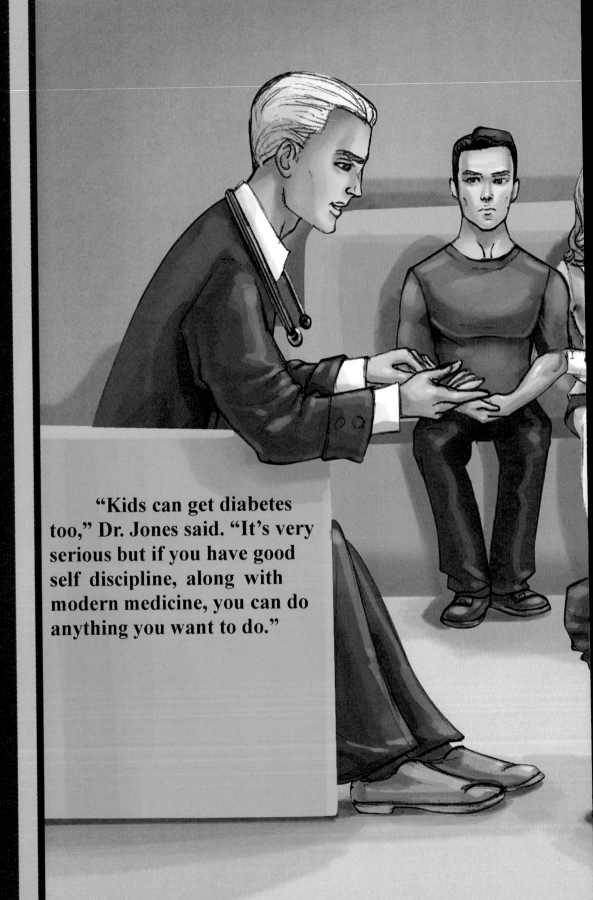

"Kids can get diabetes too," Dr. Jones said. "It's very serious but if you have good self discipline, along with modern medicine, you can do anything you want to do."

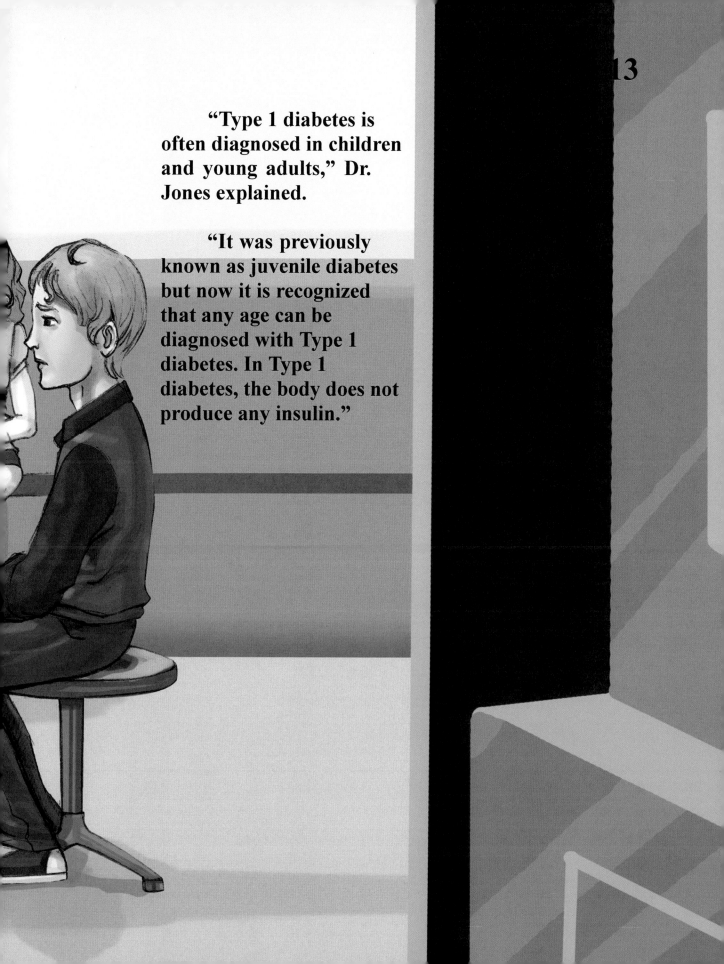

"Type 1 diabetes is often diagnosed in children and young adults," Dr. Jones explained.

"It was previously known as juvenile diabetes but now it is recognized that any age can be diagnosed with Type 1 diabetes. In Type 1 diabetes, the body does not produce any insulin."

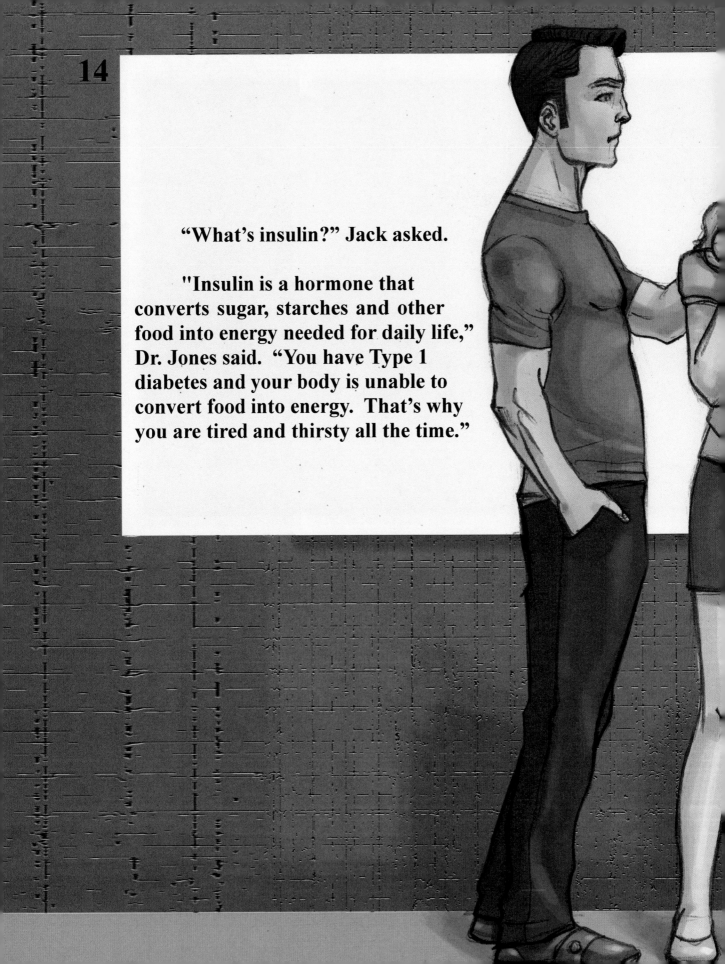

"What's insulin?" Jack asked.

"Insulin is a hormone that converts sugar, starches and other food into energy needed for daily life," Dr. Jones said. "You have Type 1 diabetes and your body is unable to convert food into energy. That's why you are tired and thirsty all the time."

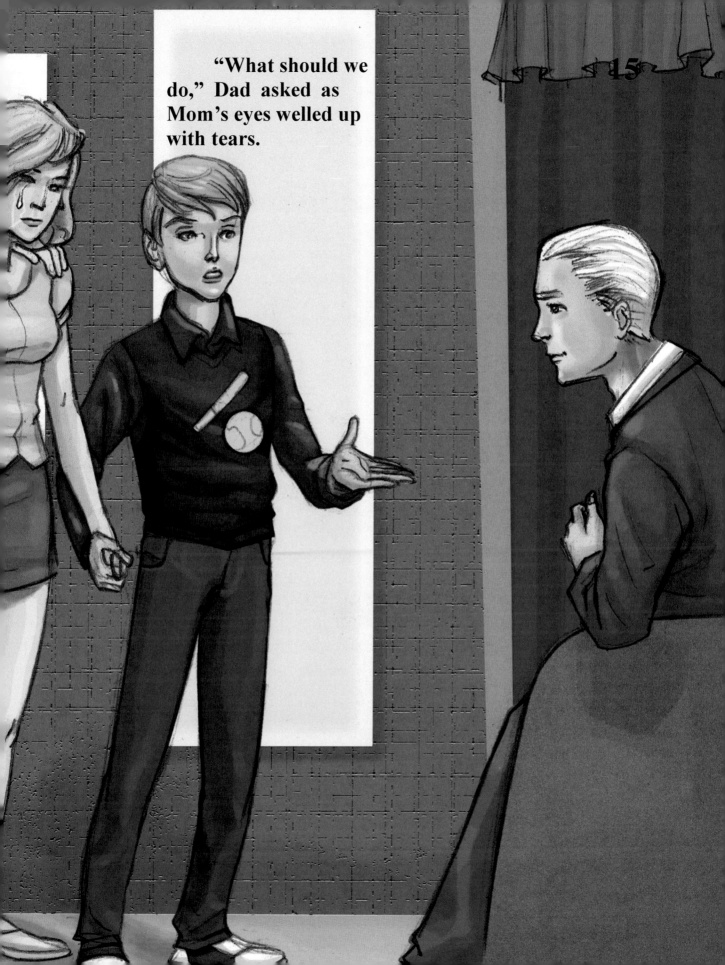

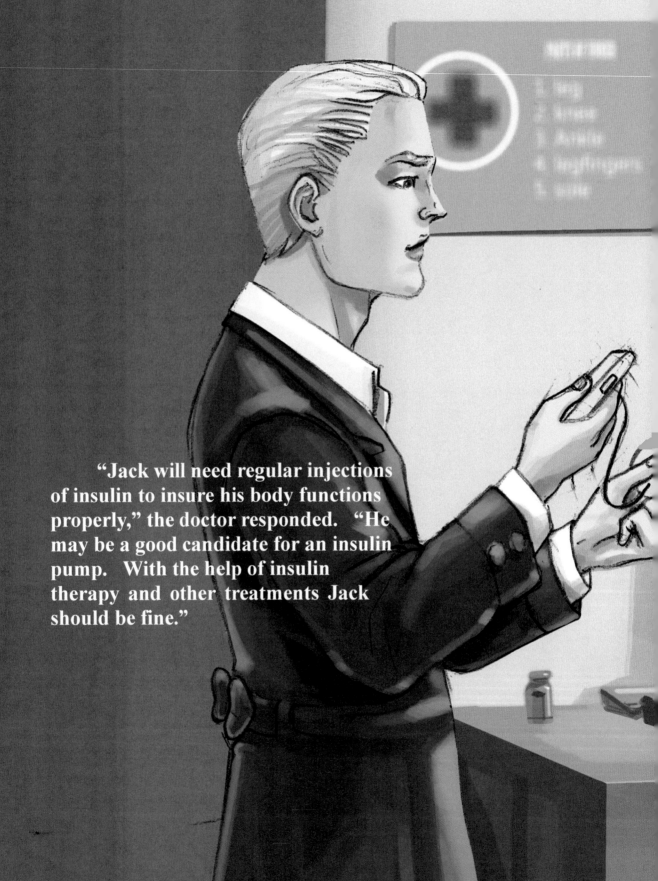

"Jack will need regular injections of insulin to insure his body functions properly," the doctor responded. "He may be a good candidate for an insulin pump. With the help of insulin therapy and other treatments Jack should be fine."

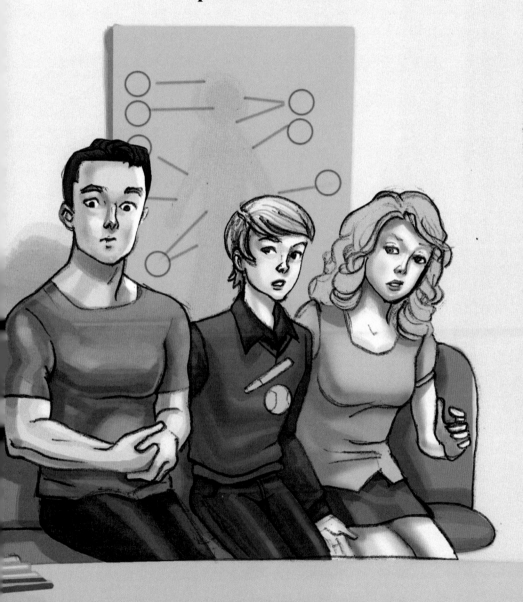

"A pump?" Jack asked.

"Yes, I think an insulin pump is less trouble than having multiple injections each day," explained Dr. Jones.

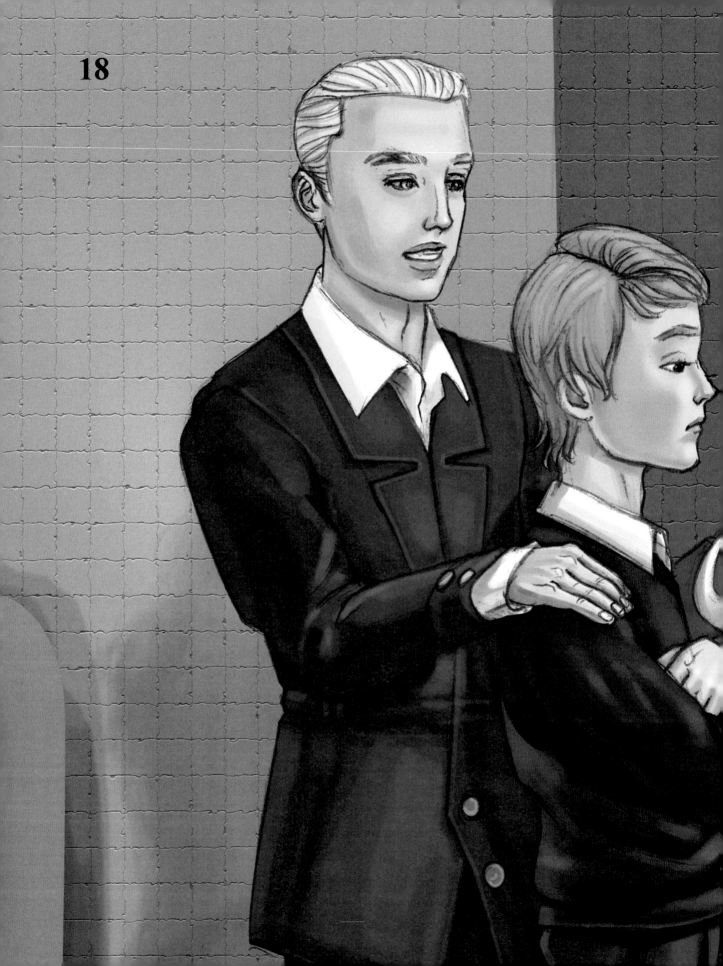

Injections? MULTIPLE injections every day? No way, thought Jack.

Seeing the look on Jack's face, Dr. Jones patted his shoulder and reassured him,

"Don't worry, Jack, it isn't as bad as it sounds.

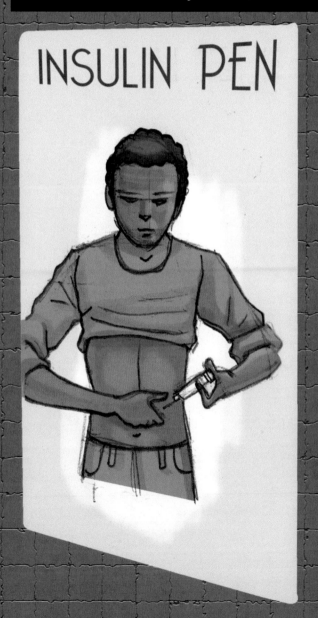

INSULIN PEN

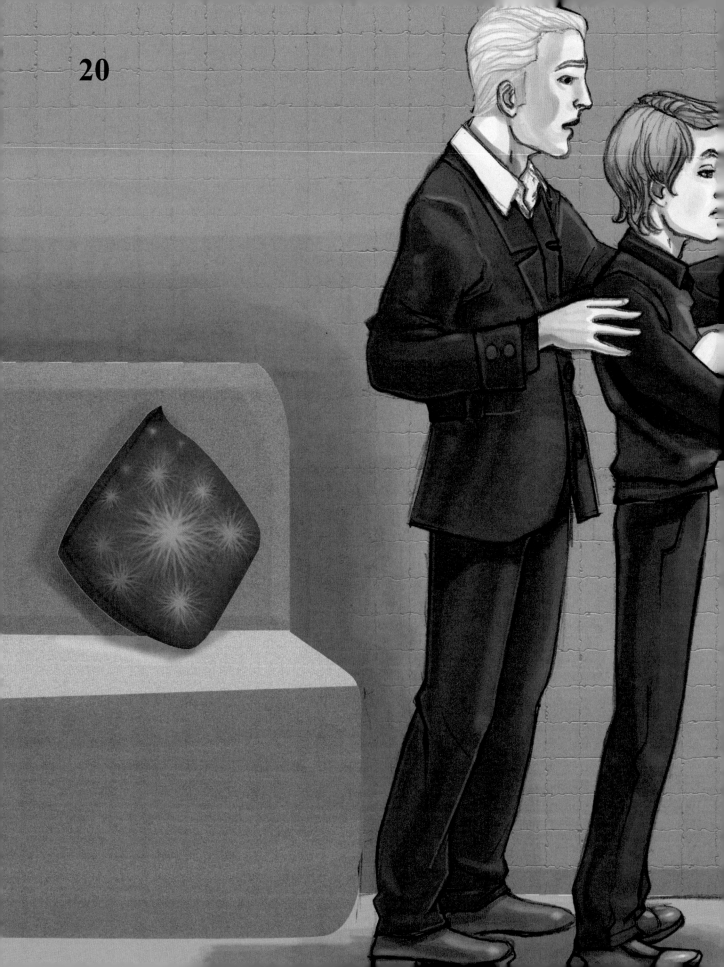

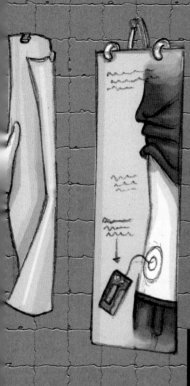

"An insulin pump is a small computerized device designed to precisely deliver insulin to the body through a small tube inserted in the skin," he explained. "Once we hook up the pump, it provides insulin as you need it and you won't need the injections every day."

Jack sighed with relief and thought, *I can handle shots; I just don't like them.*

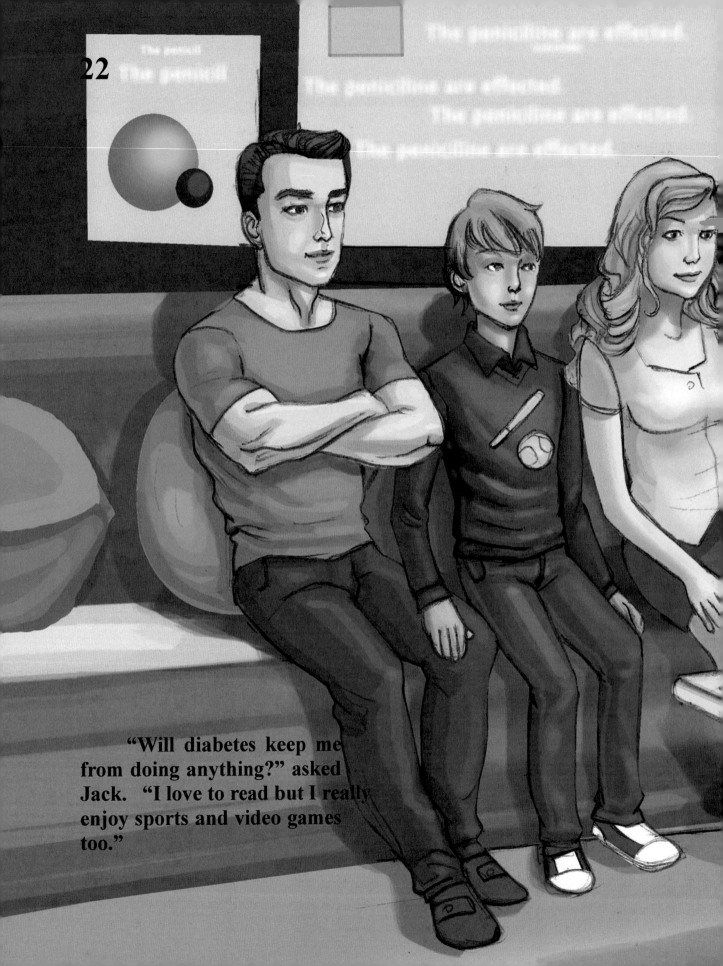

"Will diabetes keep me from doing anything?" asked Jack. "I love to read but I really enjoy sports and video games too."

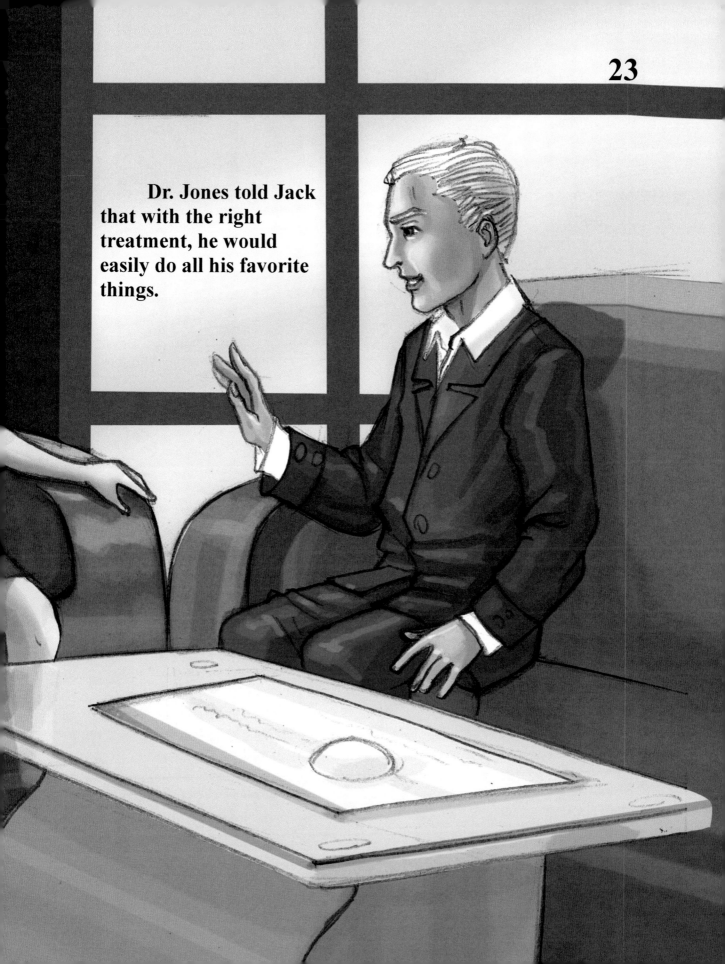

Dr. Jones told Jack that with the right treatment, he would easily do all his favorite things.

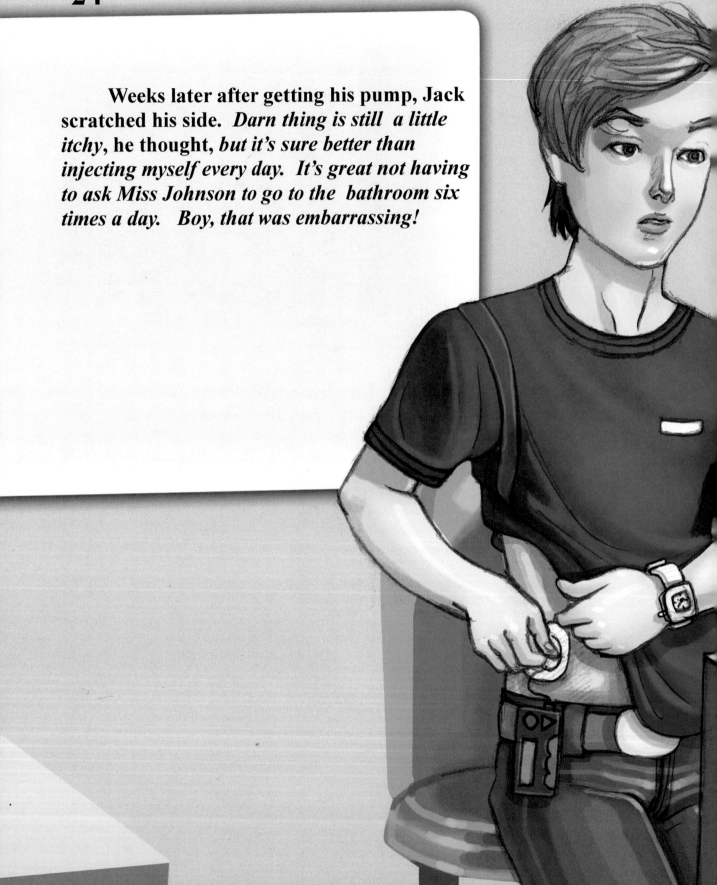

Weeks later after getting his pump, Jack scratched his side. *Darn thing is still a little itchy*, he thought, *but it's sure better than injecting myself every day. It's great not having to ask Miss Johnson to go to the bathroom six times a day. Boy, that was embarrassing!*

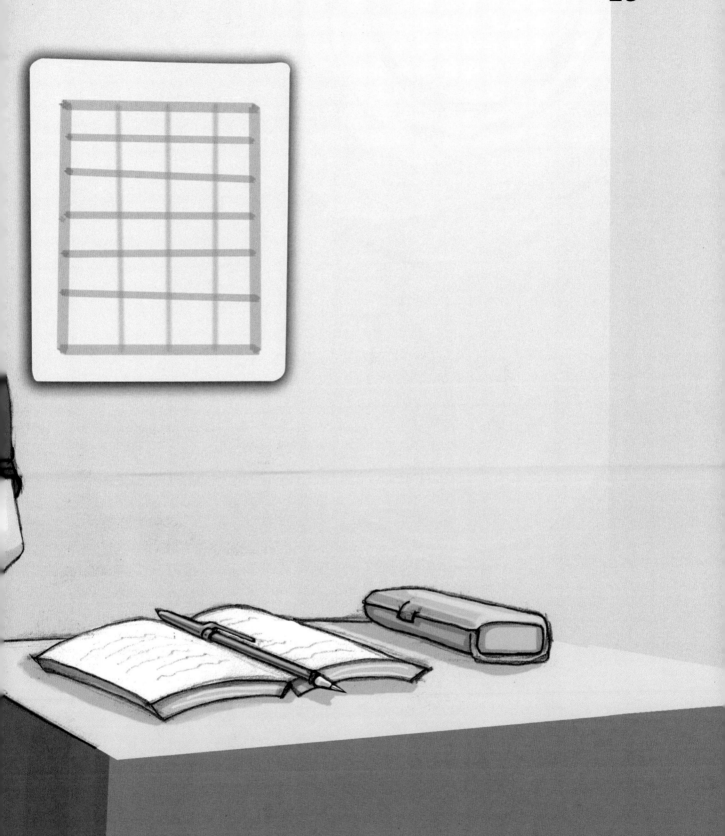

The pump is pretty cool, he thought, *but sometimes it makes a funny noise.* He laughed at himself remembering the first time the alarm went off. He freaked even though Dr. Jones

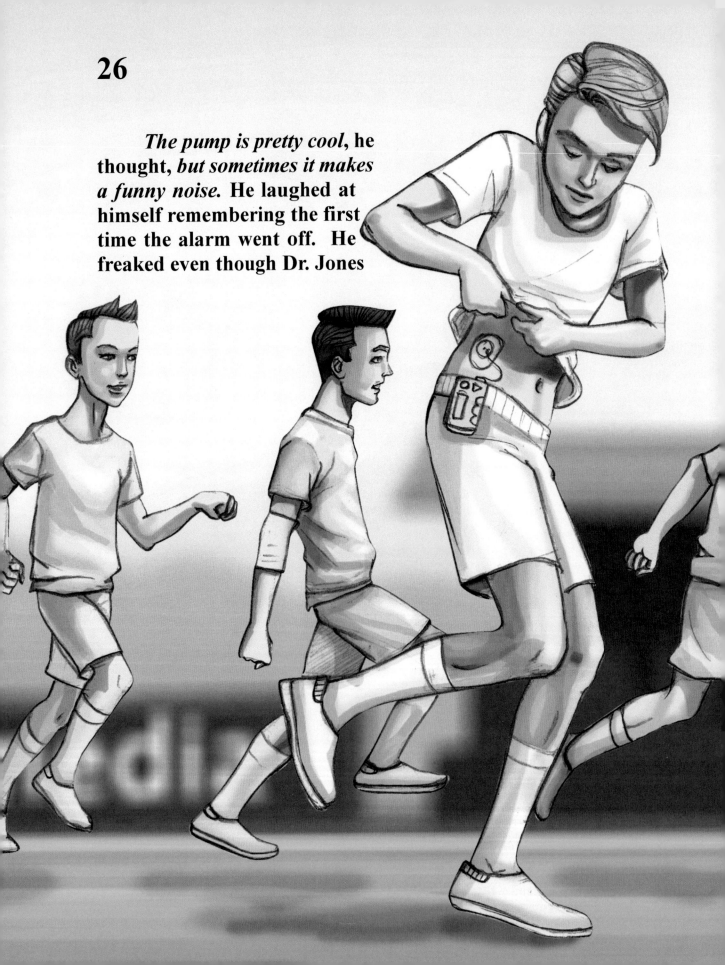

had warned him when he demonstrated how it worked. Jack liked the vibrating alarm much better than the beep. Sometimes in a capture the flag game in gym, things got way too noisy to hear a beeping. But when your side is vibrating it's hard to ignore.

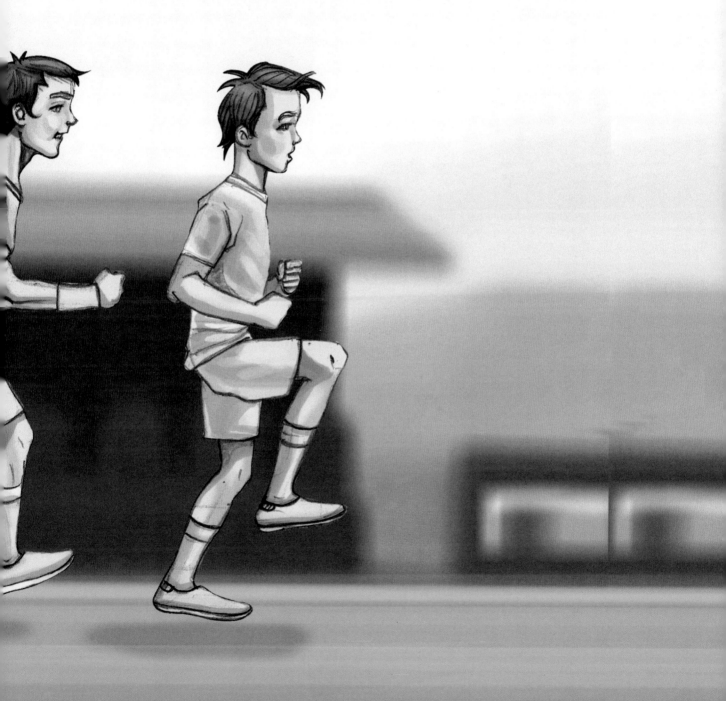

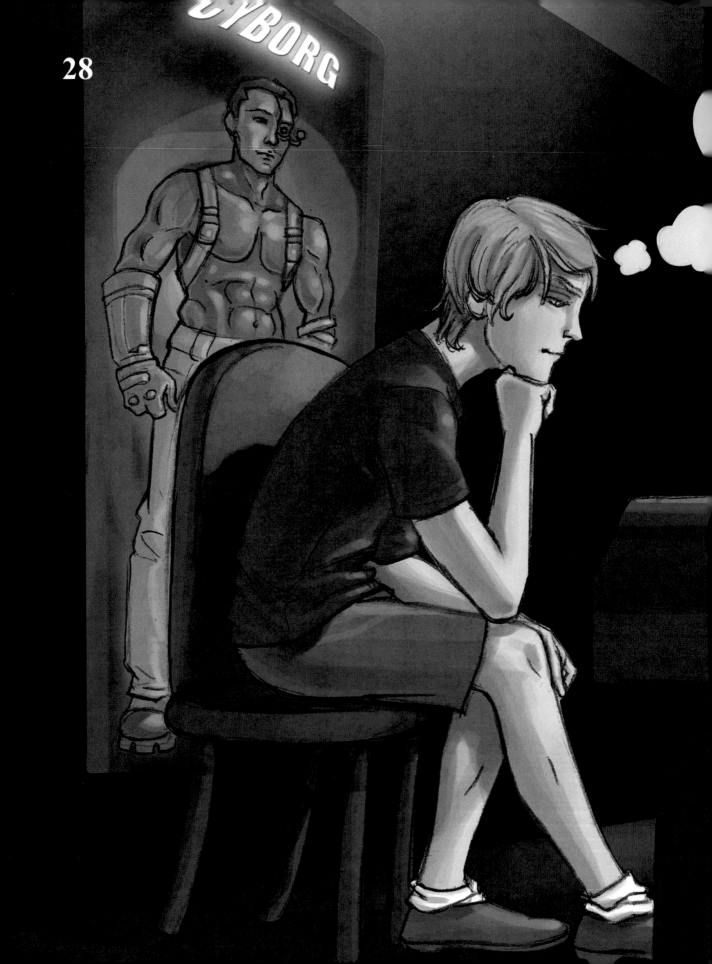

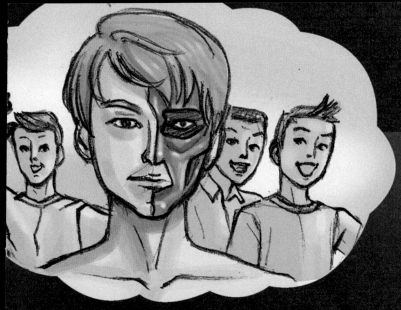

Jack figured his buddies would be
cool about the pump but he worried
about what the other kids might say.
He had wondered about cyborg
comments or gear head or if kids would
make fun of him.   Not that he couldn't
handle that but still.

"Why don't you ask Miss Johnson if you can do a science report on diabetes and the pump and show the class how cool it is," Dad had suggested. "You're a whiz at PowerPoint."

All the kids were interested in his report and loved the whole pump idea. *Well, everyone except Joey,* he thought. But nobody pays any attention to Joey anyway. Everybody knows he's just flat out rude.

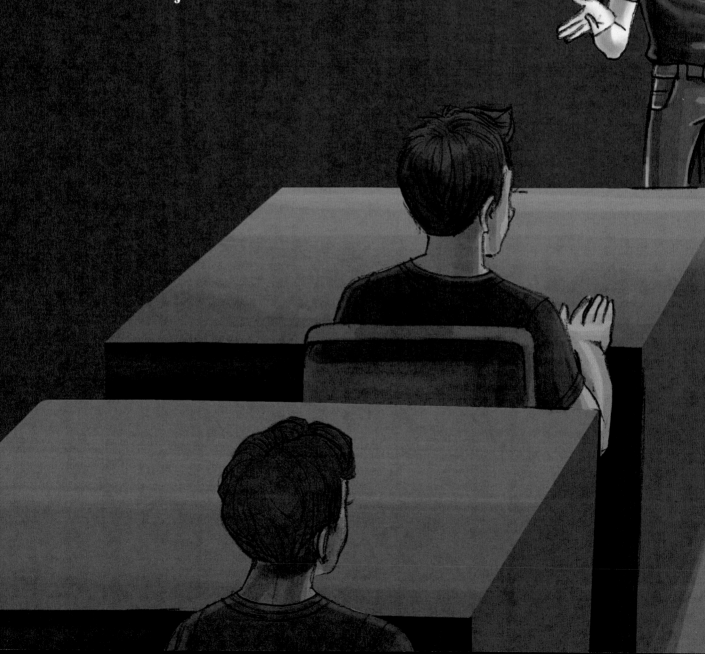

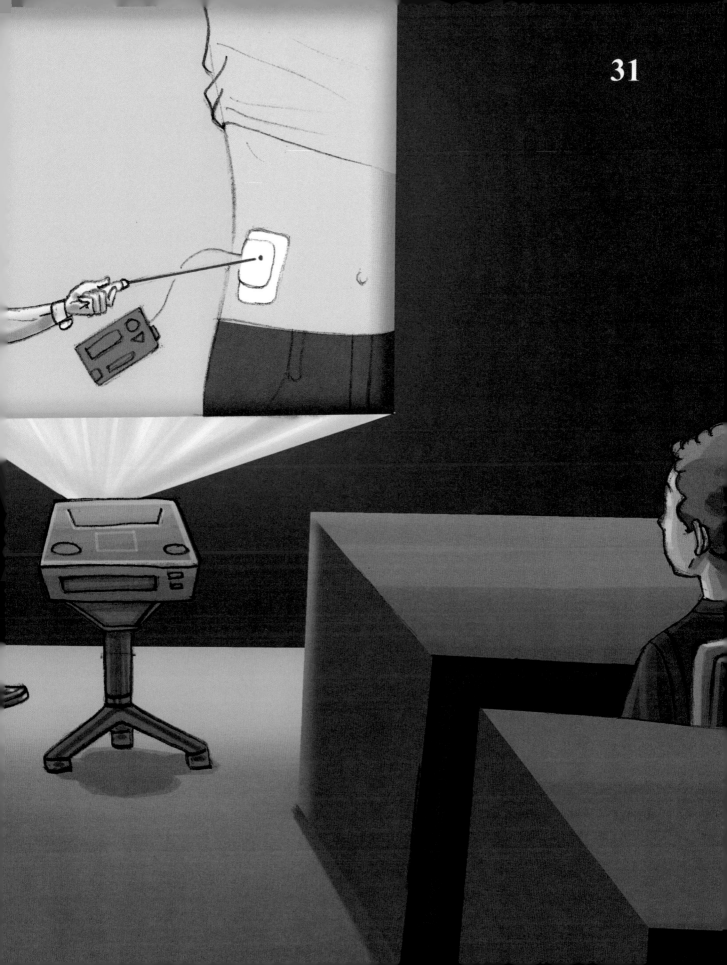

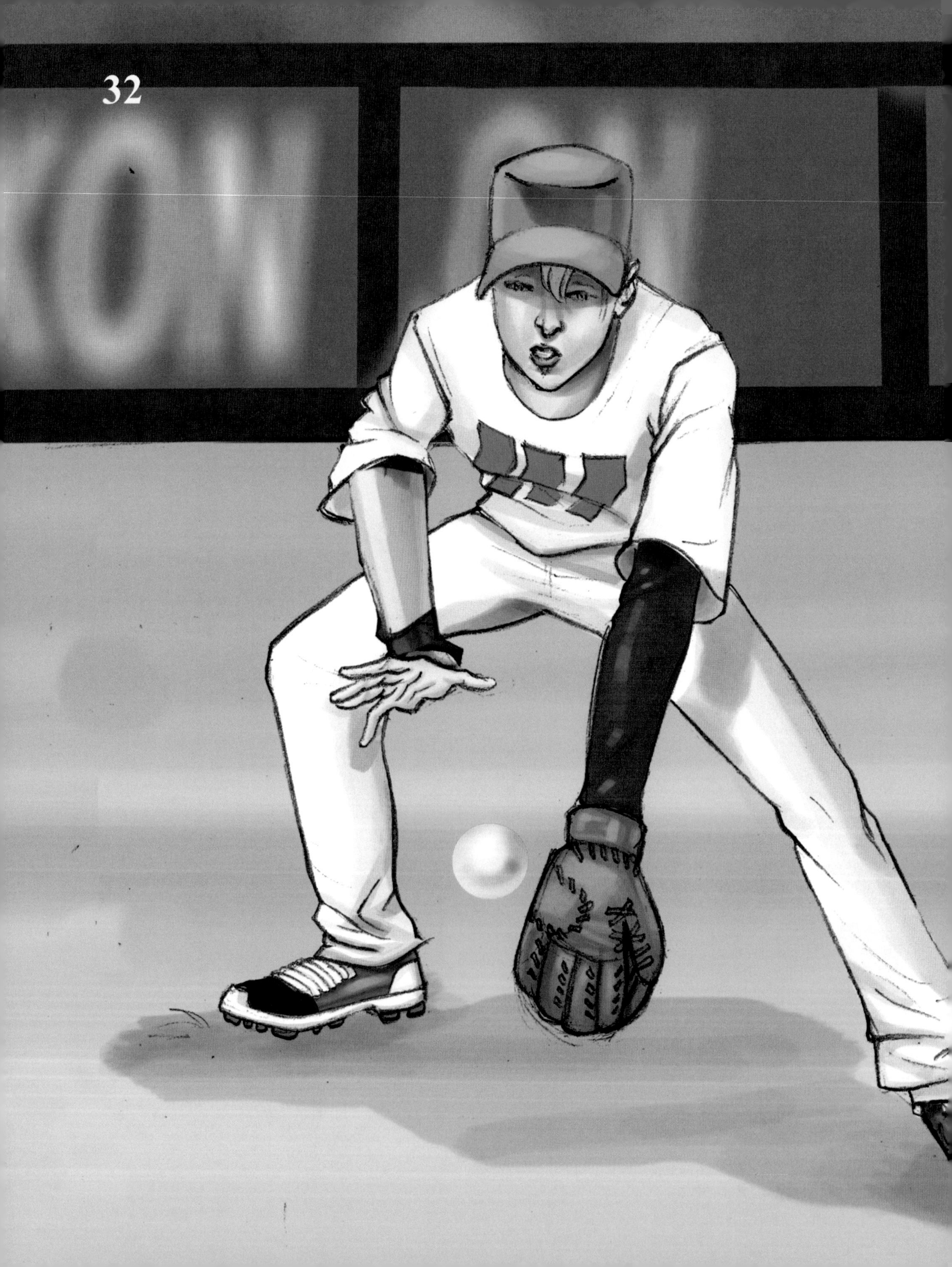

Yeah, this whole diabetes thing is pretty scary, but I have things under control, he thought to himself.

"WHACK!" A loud crack startled him out of his daydream.

A hard charging ground ball came toward him and he had to hustle to scoop it up.

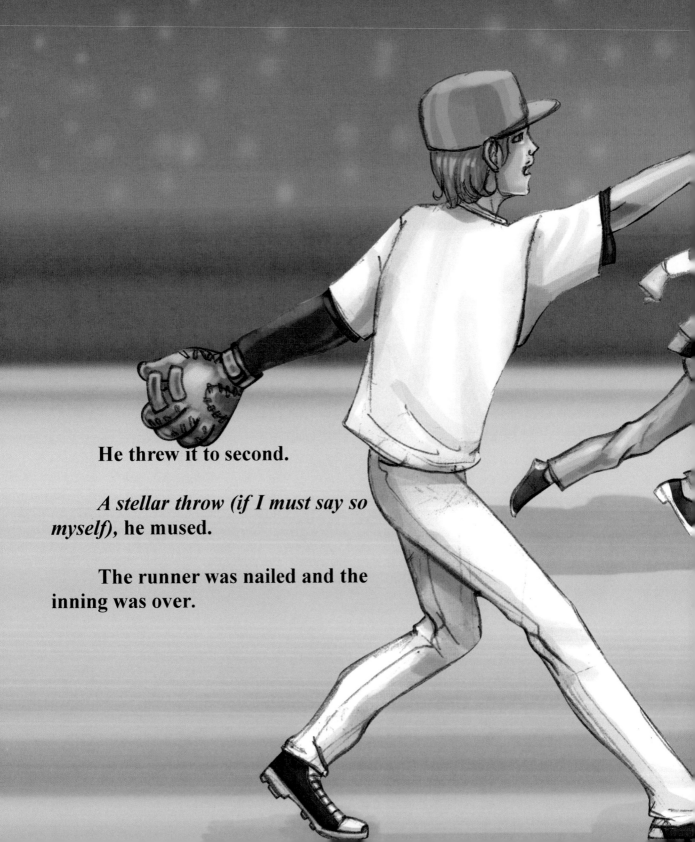

He threw it to second.

A stellar throw (if I must say so myself), he mused.

The runner was nailed and the inning was over.

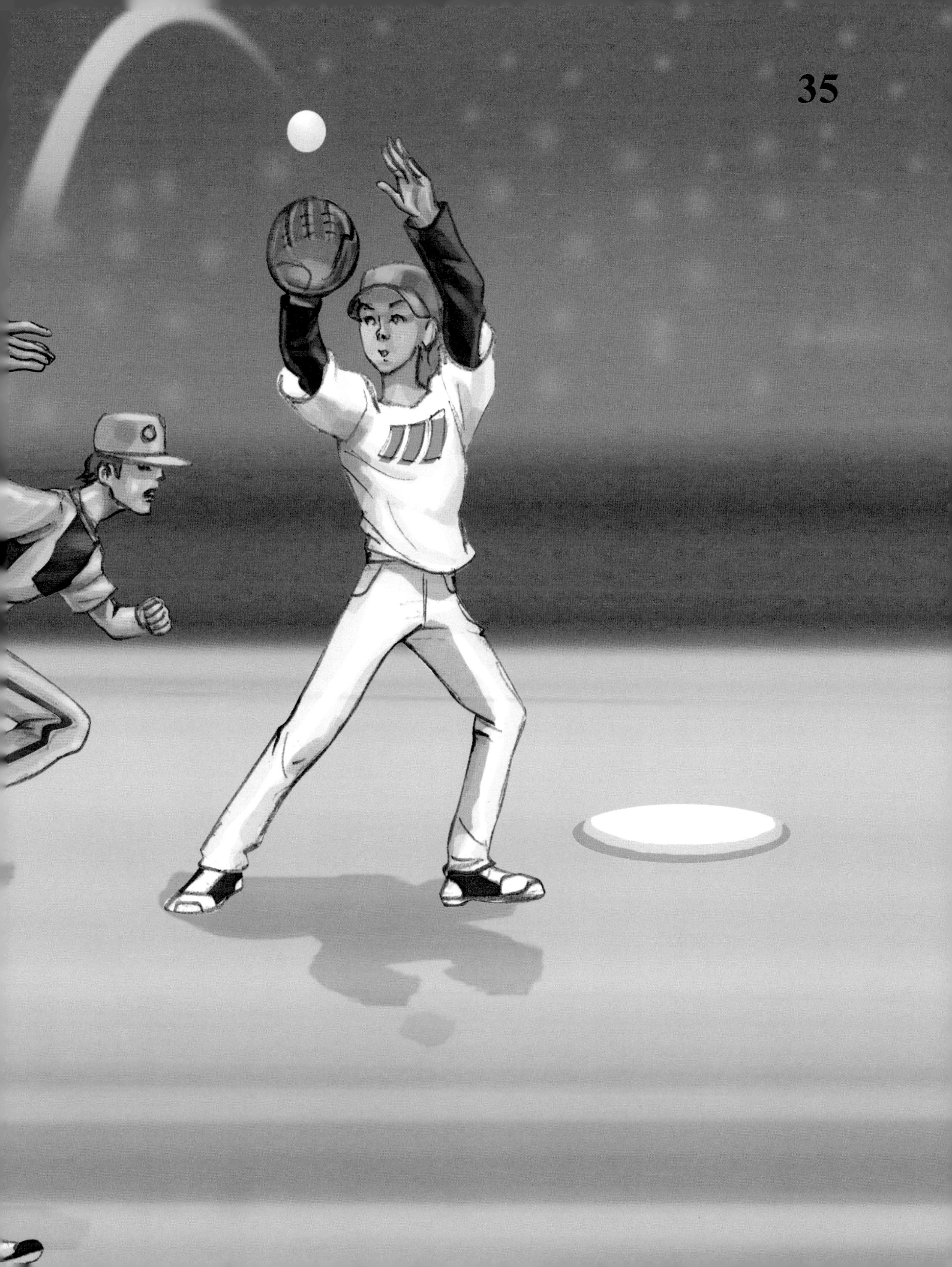

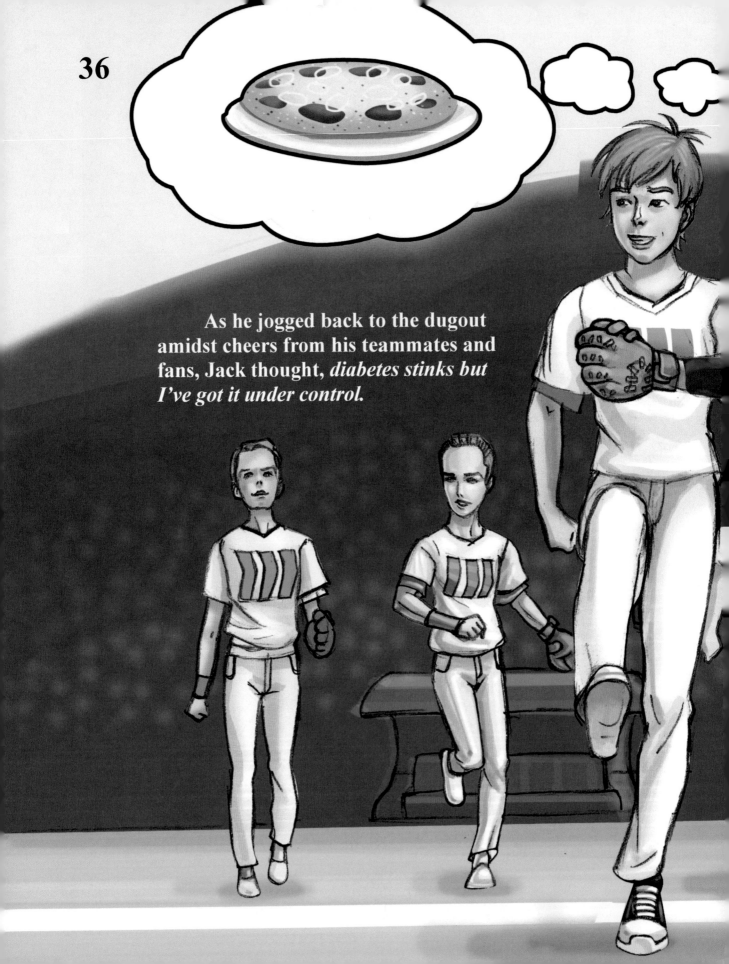

As he jogged back to the dugout amidst cheers from his teammates and fans, Jack thought, *diabetes stinks but I've got it under control.*

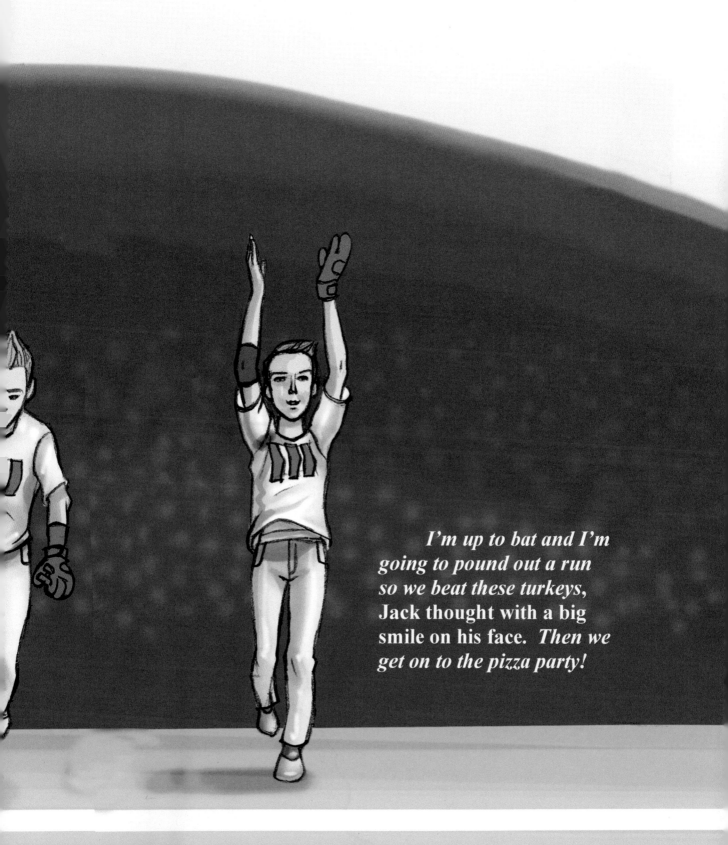

I'm up to bat and I'm going to pound out a run so we beat these turkeys, Jack thought with a big smile on his face. *Then we get on to the pizza party!*

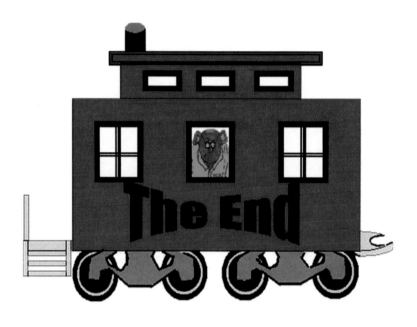

Resources

Defining of Type 1 & Type 2 Diabetes

The following definitions are taken from an ABC news website.
(http://abcnews.go.com/Health/DiabetesOverview/story?id=3843306#.T5LwS9VGw4I)

The medical professional answering the question is Steven Edelman, M.D., Professor of Medicine, Division of Endocrinology and Diabetes, University of California, San Diego
August 12, 2008
Question: What is the difference between type 1 diabetes and type 2 diabetes?

Answer: "There are several types of diabetes; I'm going to discuss the two main types: type 1 and type 2. Type 1 formerly called juvenile onset diabetes occurs typically before the age of 20. Individuals with type 1 diabetes are usually thin, and the cause of type 1 diabetes is that the pancreas, the organ that secretes insulin, is destroyed by autoantibodies, that's why people with type 1 diabetes always need insulin, either injected or through an insulin pump. Type 1 diabetes occurs in about 10-15 percent of all the diabetics in the country.

"Now, the most common type of diabetes is what we call type 2, formerly called adult onset. Type 2 diabetics are usually heavy, usually diagnosed after the age of 35. Now, the cause of type 2 diabetes is quite different from type 1. The cause of type 2 diabetes is primarily a complicated medical condition called ' insulin resistance.' In fact, in the early stages of type 2 diabetes, there's plenty of insulin around, it just doesn't work well. To treat type 2 diabetes, we typically use lifestyle, and that may work alone -- just diet and exercise -- then we may need oral medications, and it is not uncommon for someone with type 2 diabetes to eventually need insulin, either with or without the oral medications.

"Now, type 2 diabetes accounts for approximately 85 to 90 percent of all the diabetics in the country. The other important thing that needs to be said is that type 2 diabetes is associated with heart disease, and that's why it's so important to not only treat the glucose levels, but also to attack blood pressure and cholesterol levels as well. We know that type 2 diabetes runs very strongly from generation to generation, and we also know that we can prevent type 2 diabetes if we recognize it at an early stage.

"The last important thing to mention about type 1 and type 2 diabetes is that you can get any type of diabetes at any age. That's very important and that's why the American Diabetes Association changed the name from 'juvenile onset' to 'type 1,' and 'adult onset' to 'type 2.'"

Information Resources on Diabetes

National Diabetes Education Program
This website has links to a wealth of data on diabetes.

NDEP is a partnership of the National Institutes of Health, the Centers for Disease Control and Prevention, and more than 200 public and private organizations.
http://ndep.nih.gov/resources/

Health Information Phone Lines
U. S. Department of Health & Human Services National Institutes of Health
Diabetes Information   888-693-6337
National Diabetes Education Program   800-438-5383

American Diabetes Association: Diabetes Hotline
Information provided by Santa Clara Valley Health & Hospital System / Mental Health Department.
Phone line provides information and referrals regarding diabetes.
Phone Number:(800) 828-8293

DiabetesDaily.com – an online community for people with diabetes
http://www.diabetesdaily.com/

JDRF formerly known as the Juvenile Diabetes Research Foundation is known simply as JDRF since 85 percent of those in the U.S with type 1 diabetes are adults.
 http://www.jdrf.org/

Please note that I'm not a medical professional and these information sources are only provided as a courtesy, I am not endorsing or recommending any of them.

http://diabetes.emedtv.com/insulin-pumps/insulin-pump-warnings-and-precautions.html

http://www.mayoclinic.com/health/type-1-diabetes-in-children/DS00931/DSECTION=symptoms

http://www.diabetes.org/diabetes-basics/type-1/

Other Books By Author William G. Bentrim That You May Enjoy.

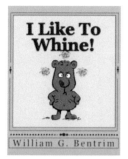

I Like To Whine is a series of scenarios of animals whining and the wise old owl gently chiding them and making suggestions as to why whining is inappropriate. At the end of the book there are some parenting strategies and activities for dealing with whining children. It is focused on elementary age children.
ISBN-10: 1442131721
ISBN-13: 978-1442131729

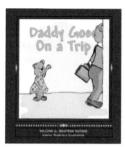

Daddy Goes On A Trip addresses pre-school children and their concerns about parents who travel or are **deployed.** It is focused on elementary age children. At the end of the book there are some parenting strategies and activities for dealing with the stresses of military deployment and parental travel.
ISBN-10: 1449539734
ISBN-13: 978-1449539733

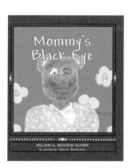

Mommy's Black Eye is a children's book that addresses the complicated issue of domestic violence. It is focused on pre-school to middle school children. At the end of the book there are some parenting strategies and activities for dealing with this complicated issue.   There are helpful contacts for those who find themselves in a domestic violence situation.
ISBN-10: 1449512577   **Also in Kindle Format**
ISBN-13: 978-1449512576
Also see El ojo morado de Mama (Spanish Edition)

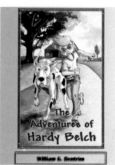

The Adventures of Hardy Belch is a chapter book that chronicles the exciting and unbelievable adventures of a 12-year-old boy and his 240-pound telepathic dog. In this book, Hardy copes with a bully, learns about intolerance and discovers the value of community cooperation. Parent resources on bullying and intolerance are included. Combining mystery and humor each story is written to entertain and highlight the value of friendship, planning and selfless actions.
ISBN-10: 1449918530
ISBN-13: 978-1449918538

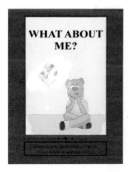

What About Me? This book looks at the feelings that siblings of injured or sick children face daily. Often parents overlook the impact on all their children of overt focusing on a child that may be injured or ill. Older children can normally deal with this through logical thought, younger children frequently react emotionally. Hopefully, this book will help the younger child understand and deal with his or her feelings.
ISBN-10: 1451547927
ISBN-13: 978-1451547924

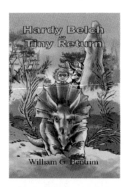

Hardy Belch and Tiny Return Hardy Belch, a 12-year-old boy, and Tiny, his 240-pound telepathic dog, return in their second book. Hardy and Tiny find themselves facing a paleontologist's dream, a disappearing train and the infamous Bucks County Pennsylvania Doan gang of notorious outlaws in this book. The secret of how Tiny got his telepathic ability is also revealed. Hardy and Tiny have a rollicking good time while helping others. Combining mystery and humor each story is written to entertain and highlight the value of friendship, planning and selfless actions.

ISBN-10: 1449930883   ISBN-13: 978-1449930882

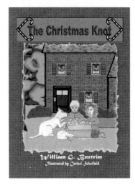

The Christmas Knot is a delightful tale of two kids and a puppy named Tiny. The three find themselves wrapped up in a knotty problem. Working with their parents they are able to untangle their problem and contribute to the spirit of the season. The story features a very young Hardy Belch, his cousin Mardi and his puppy Tiny. Hardy and Tiny are the main characters in the Hardy Belch chapter books.

ISBN-10: 1453701060   Also in Kindle Format
ISBN-13: 978-1453701065

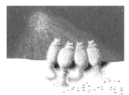

A Quirky Christmas Quirky is a red-tailed, grey squirrel with an adventurous nature and a huge heart. Quirky and his friends, Stubby and Art, help Reggie, a selfish squirrel, discover the meaning of friendship, sharing and the beauty of Christmas.

ISBN-13: 978-1456474379   Also in Kindle Format
ISBN-10: 1456474375

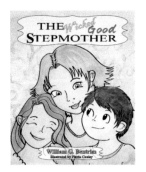

The Wicked Good Stepmother Bonnie and Bradley's mother passed away several years ago. While their father is deployed he meets a woman, falls in love and gets married. Now he is coming home with his new wife who is now his children's stepmother. Bonnie and Bradley know all about how wicked stepmothers are from their story books. They are scared to death to meet their new mom. What happens when they meet the ***Wicked Good Stepmother***?

ISBN-13: 978-1452839462   Also in Kindle Format
ISBN-10: 1452839468

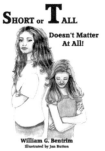

Short or Tall, Doesn't Matter At All

Elisabeth is the shortest girl in 5th grade and often the target of bullies. She proves to herself and to her peers that how tall you are doesn't define who you are.

ISBN-10: 1475082665   Also in Kindle Format
ISBN-13: 978-1475082661

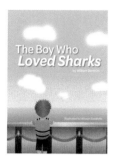

The Boy Who Loved Sharks

We have all known children that become "experts" on things they like and we have been amazed at how much they can learn when they are internally motivated. This boy is an example of how one can succeed in his dreams by using what he has learned and demonstrating his compassionate nature.

ISBN-10: 147834458X   **Also in Kindle Format**

ISBN-13: 978-1478344582

Available In Kindle Only Editions

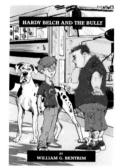

Hardy Belch And The Bully

Hardy Belch, is a normal 12 year old boy, and Tiny, his 240 pound telepathic dog is anything but normal. Bullying is a hot topic today but it has been around for generations. This story is a lighthearted look at a bully and how he is thwarted. Each story is written to entertain and highlight the values of friendship, planning and selfless actions.

ASIN: B009NSH1CU

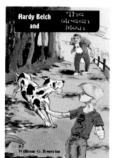

Hardy Belch and The Green Man (The Adventures of Hardy Belch)

This story has its roots in a popular Western Pennsylvania urban legend. Reality is most often stranger than fiction and this tale is a blending of both. Hardy Belch finds that fear of the unknown may lead to prejudice and intolerance. He discovers the error of his ways with the able assistance of Tiny who shares the encompassing good nature of man's best friend.

ASIN: B00CKS8QVU

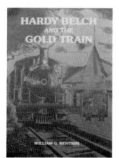

Hardy Belch and The Gold Train (The Adventures of Hardy Belch)

A mysterious, missing gold train provides a treasure hunt for Tiny and Hardy. Over one hundred years after a gold train goes missing, Hardy and Tiny find themselves knee deep in swamp muck trying to help a friend save his farm.

ASIN: B00D9UR9KM

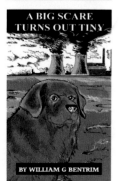

A Big Scare Turns Out Tiny (The Adventures of Hardy Belch)

This story relates the birth of 240 pound Tiny and how he may have obtained his unique characteristics. Hardy is only mentioned by name and has not joined his best friend in this story. Tiny's Mom is the heroine of this tale.

ASIN: B009NU3JCO

Made in the USA
Middletown, DE
20 January 2020

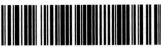